Vascular Dementia Therapy & Management

Beyond Forgetfulness, Navigating the Journey
of Vascular Cognitive Impairment.

Title:
Vascular Dementia Therapy & Management

Subtitle
Beyond Forgetfulness, Navigating the Journey of Vascular Cognitive Impairment.

Printed in the United States of America.

ISBN: 9798878418157

TABLE OF CONTENT

INTRODUCTION

Vascular dementia is a neurodegenerative condition that is defined by cognitive deterioration as a result of reduced blood flow to the brain. It ranks among the most serious challenges that might be encountered in the field of neurodegenerative disorders. We must delve deeply into the fundamental aspects that lay the groundwork for understanding this condition and its nuances as we embark on the exploration of Vascular Dementia Therapy and Management. This is because doing so will lay the foundation for our understanding of the condition.

Definition and Overview of Vascular Dementia

Vascular dementia, also known as post-stroke dementia, is a state of cognitive impairment brought on by diminished blood supply to the brain as a result of cerebrovascular illnesses and other ailments. Vascular dementia, in contrast to some other types of dementia, is a phrase that refers to a group of cognitive illnesses that have similar vascular origins.

Cerebrovascular disease, which is frequently the consequence of strokes or other disorders affecting the blood arteries in the brain, causes the cognitive decline associated with vascular dementia. Sometimes, a range of cognitive abnormalities brought on by vascular factors—

from moderate cognitive impairment to severe dementia—are referred to as "vascular cognitive impairment."

Comprehending the many classifications of vascular dementia is crucial in customizing efficacious treatment approaches. Among the other classifications are subcortical vascular dementia, multi-infarct dementia, and strategic infarct dementia, each of which presents unique clinical characteristics. Vascular risk factors, including diabetes, atherosclerosis, and hypertension, interact to form the complex pathophysiology of this disease.

Vascular dementia affects memory, executive function, and day-to-day activities, influencing a broad range of cognitive and functional deficits. The diagnostic approach is made more difficult by the possibility of cognitive changes in people with vascular dementia. It is crucial to understand that vascular dementia can coexist with other types of dementia, such as Alzheimer's disease, which can make the clinical picture even more challenging.

Prevalence and Incidence

Vascular risk factors, age, and ethnicity all have an impact on the changing epidemiological picture of vascular dementia. Vascular dementia is widely regarded as the second most prevalent cause of dementia after Alzheimer's disease, but incidence varies among various populations.

Vascular dementia is more common as people age, with people over 65 having a greater frequency of the condition. Vascular dementia and age have a complex association that is influenced throughout time by the cumulative effects of vascular risk factors. Interestingly, vascular dementia frequently coexists with other age-related illnesses, highlighting the necessity of complete geriatric treatment.

Geographic differences in vascular dementia prevalence highlight the impact of lifestyle, environmental, and genetic variables. Vascular dementia is more common in areas where vascular risk factors, such as smoking, a sedentary lifestyle, and poor nutrition, are more common. Identifying these trends is essential to creating focused public health initiatives that lessen the effects of vascular dementia on local populations.

Importance of Early Diagnosis

For afflicted people and their families, early detection of vascular dementia is essential to improving outcomes and raising quality of life. Vascular dementia manifests differently from certain other types of dementia in that it frequently occurs suddenly and progresses gradually. This means that early detection is essential to the implementation of therapies.

Early diagnosis is critical for more than just managing symptoms; it also affects treating underlying vascular causes and halting further cognitive impairment. Neuroimaging and neuropsychological testing are two important diagnostic tools that are used to confirm the diagnosis and differentiate vascular dementia from other cognitive diseases.

Healthcare providers can create individualized treatment regimens with both pharmaceutical and non-pharmacological tactics when early intervention is used. Antihypertensive and antiplatelet medications, among others, that target vascular risk factors may help to halt the course of vascular dementia. Additionally, interventions like as caregiver support, cognitive rehabilitation, and lifestyle adjustments are more successful when started early in the disease.

From a social standpoint, early diagnosis makes healthcare system planning and resource allocation easier. It makes it possible to create community activities, education campaigns, and support services targeted at increasing knowledge of vascular dementia and lessening its stigma.

UNDERSTANDING VASCULAR DEMENTIA

As we get deeper into the center of our investigation on Vascular Dementia Therapy and Management, we must have a solid understanding of the complexities that lie behind this disorder. To gain an understanding of vascular dementia, it is necessary to investigate its contributing factors and causes, to investigate the pathophysiology that governs the progression of the disease, and to differentiate between the various types of dementia that manifest with different clinical characteristics.

Causes and Risk Factors

- **Vascular Risk Factors:**

Numerous vascular risk factors are closely linked to vascular dementia, and these variables collectively contribute to the complex mosaic of cerebrovascular disorders. The delicate cerebral arteries are subjected to constant pressure from hypertension, a major contributor to vascular injury, which increases their vulnerability to harm. The artery walls are gradually weakened by prolonged exposure to high blood pressure, which opens the door for the formation of microinfarcts and ischemic lesions that are indicative of vascular dementia.

Another serious risk factor is diabetes mellitus, a metabolic disease marked by poor management of blood glucose. The cerebral vasculature is further compromised by systemic inflammation and endothelial dysfunction brought on by the persistent hyperglycemia linked to diabetes. The complex interaction of oxidative stress, inflammation, and insulin resistance fosters vascular disease and accelerates cognitive decline.

Smoking is a modifiable risk factor that increases the bloodstream's concentration of several toxic chemicals that cause vascular inflammation and atherosclerosis. Nicotine, carbon monoxide, and other harmful substances work together to hasten blood vessel constriction, which reduces blood supply to the brain. Quitting smoking is a crucial intervention in the management and prevention of vascular dementia, highlighting the need to change one's lifestyle.

- **Atherosclerosis and Cerebrovascular Diseases:**

Vascular dementia is mostly caused by atherosclerosis, which is defined as the buildup of plaque in arteries. The cholesterol, inflammatory cells, and cellular debris that make up atheromatous plaques block blood arteries, preventing the brain from receiving oxygen and nutrition. Severe occurrences of atherosclerotic plaque rupture can result in embolism and thrombosis, which set off ischemia events that ultimately impair cognitive function.

Vascular dementia has a strong etiology that includes a range of disorders affecting the blood arteries in the brain. These disorders are known as cerebrovascular illnesses. Ischemic strokes can lead to localized neurological impairments and cognitive dysfunction because they are caused by cerebral artery blockage. A unique set of difficulties arises from hemorrhagic strokes, which are defined by bleeding inside the brain parenchyma and frequently result in abrupt and severe cognitive deterioration.

- **Genetic Factors and Vascular Dementia:**

Genetic predisposition influences susceptibility to cerebrovascular disorders, even if acquired risk factors are the main cause of vascular dementia. A person's chance of acquiring vascular dementia is influenced by certain genetic variants and familial clustering of vascular risk factors. There is potential for finding new therapy targets and improving risk prediction models by investigating the genetic foundations of this illness.

Pathophysiology of Vascular Dementia

- **Ischemic Cascade:**

An ischemic cascade, which is the pathophysiology of vascular dementia, is typified by an inadequate blood supply to the brain that sets off a sequence of events that ultimately result in neuronal damage and cognitive impairment. Excitatory neurotransmitters are released in excess during ischemia, which causes calcium ions to flood neurons. A series of intracellular processes, such as the production of free radicals and the activation of proteases, are triggered by this calcium excess and ultimately lead to neuronal death.

16

Vascular dementia is characterized by chronic hypoperfusion, which aggravates the ischemic cascade and prolongs neuronal dysfunction. Because of the impaired cerebral blood flow, harmful metabolites are more difficult to remove from the body and vital nutrients are not delivered, which creates an environment that is favorable to neurodegeneration. White matter lesions, frequently seen in neuroimaging examinations of patients suffering from vascular dementia, are indicative of the cumulative damage that persistent ischemia has done to the structural integrity of the brain.

- **Microvascular Changes:**

The etiology of vascular dementia is largely dependent on microvascular pathology, with small vessel dysfunction emerging as a common denominator. A variety of pathological alterations, such as microinfarcts, lipo hyalinosis, and arteriolosclerosis, are included in small vessel disease and all contribute to cognitive decline. The autoregulation of cerebral blood flow is disrupted by the arteriolar alterations, leaving the brain susceptible to variations in blood pressure.

Small patches of ischemia damage dispersed throughout the brain, known as cerebral microinfarcts, have drawn attention as one of the main causes of cognitive impairment in vascular dementia. These silent infarcts gradually build up and affect cognitive function cumulatively. They are frequently undetectable on conventional neuroimaging. The crucial role that microinfarcts play in the development of vascular dementia is further highlighted by their strategic placement inside important brain networks.

- **Blood-Brain Barrier Dysfunction:**

Vascular dementia compromises the integrity of the blood-brain barrier (BBB), a dynamic interface that controls the flow of chemicals between the circulation and the brain. Inflammatory mediators can enter the brain parenchyma through the disruption of tight connections between endothelial cells caused by oxidative stress and chronic inflammation brought on by vascular risk factors. Failure of the BBB increases neuroinflammation, makes it easier for immune cells to infiltrate, and increases the risk of neuronal damage.

Developing focused therapy strategies is made possible by having a framework for understanding the pathophysiological causes of vascular dementia. Vascular pathology is complex and requires a multimodal strategy that addresses both the microscopic and macroscopic alterations that cause cognitive loss.

Types of Vascular Dementia

- **Subcortical Vascular Dementia:**

Binswanger's illness, commonly referred to as subcortical vascular dementia, largely damages the brain's white matter. This subtype is characterized by a large amount of damage to the tiny capillaries that supply subcortical areas. It also manifests as motor abnormalities, emotional disorders, and cognitive deficiencies. White matter hyperintensities and lacunar infarcts are characteristic neuroimaging results that indicate extensive ischemia alterations within the subcortical areas.

- **Multi-infarct Dementia:**

The cumulative effects of several little infarcts across the brain, which are frequently brought on by embolic or thrombotic events, are what define multi-infarct dementia. Distinctive from other types of dementia is the sudden onset and progressive nature of cognitive impairments in multi-infarct dementia. Dispersed infarcts in various vascular areas are shown by neuroimaging investigations, which may account for the varied clinical presentation seen in afflicted people.

- **Strategic Infarct Dementia:**

Distinct infarcts in certain brain areas that are essential for cognitive function are linked to strategic infarct dementia. Significant cognitive damage can result from infarcts that occur in key areas, such as the thalamus or angular gyrus. Often, specific neurological impairments matching the infarct's site characterize the clinical presentation. The relevance of lesion placement in defining the cognitive profile of patients with vascular dementia is underscored by strategic infarct dementia.

DIAGNOSTIC APPROACHES

The quick and accurate identification of vascular dementia is a crucial cornerstone as we traverse the complex world of vascular dementia therapy and management. Vascular dementia is diagnosed using a variety of methods, including clinical evaluation, cognitive testing, neuroimaging, and the investigation of blood-based biomarkers. Healthcare providers must have a thorough awareness of these diagnostic techniques to offer patients with vascular dementia tailored therapies and support.

Clinical Assessment and Neuropsychological Testing

- **Clinical Assessment:**

The first and most important step in the diagnosis process for vascular dementia is clinical examination. A complete medical history is part of a comprehensive examination, which also encompasses vascular risk factor assessment, including diabetes, hypertension, history of smoking, and atherosclerosis. A vascular etiology may be indicated by a rapid or gradual decline in cognitive function, which the physician looks for as they attempt to comprehend the beginning and course of cognitive symptoms.

A physical examination may identify isolated neurological impairments or abnormalities in gait as indicators of cerebrovascular illness. Evaluating the functional status and activities of daily living (ADLs) of the individual provides important information about how cognitive impairment affects day-to-day functioning. It is important to keep an eye out for mood disorders, such as sadness or apathy, as these frequently occur with vascular dementia and influence the overall clinical presentation.

- **Neuropsychological Testing:**

Since neuropsychological testing offers objective assessments of cognitive performance in a variety of domains, it is essential to the diagnostic process. Memory, executive function, attention, language, and visuospatial skills are all assessed using cognitive assessment instruments. Two widely used screening instruments that are useful for measuring cognitive deficiencies and monitoring improvements over time are the Montreal Cognitive Assessment (MoCA) and the Mini-Mental State Examination (MMSE).

Certain types of cognitive impairment that indicate the involvement of subcortical regions may appear in vascular dementia. A person may have deficiencies in executive functioning, attention span, and processing speed in addition to the memory-centric presentation that is frequently associated with Alzheimer's disease. Neuropsychological testing helps distinguish vascular dementia from other cognitive problems and establishes a baseline for tracking the course of the illness and the effectiveness of therapy.

Neuroimaging Techniques

- **Structural Imaging:**

Confirming the diagnosis of vascular dementia and explaining the underlying anatomical alterations in the brain are made possible in large part by neuroimaging. The structure of the brain may be seen in great detail thanks to structural imaging methods like computed tomography (CT) scans and magnetic resonance imaging (MRI). These pictures may show signs of cerebrovascular disease, such as microbleeds, white matter hyperintensities (WMH), and infarcts, in cases of vascular dementia.

In vascular dementia, infarcts—visible as regions of tissue damage from ischemia—are often seen. Their distribution and position can provide information about the vascular dementia subtype since many infarct patterns or strategic infarcts suggest distinct pathophysiological processes. The persistent consequences of small artery disease on the white matter pathways are reflected in WMH, which is frequently observed in subcortical vascular dementia.

- **Functional Imaging:**

Single-photon emission computed tomography (SPECT) and positron emission tomography (PET) are two functional imaging methods that offer important insights into brain blood flow and metabolic activity. These modalities provide insights into the functional effects of vascular disease by assisting in the identification of areas of hypoperfusion or hypometabolism.

Deficits in cerebral perfusion linked to vascular dementia may not always line up spatially with anatomical irregularities. This knowledge gap is filled in part by functional imaging, which offers a more thorough comprehension of the hemodynamic alterations linked to vascular dementia. When combined with structural imaging, functional imaging improves diagnostic precision and helps distinguish vascular dementia from other neurodegenerative conditions.

- **Amyloid Imaging:**

Vascular dementia can occur in conjunction with other types of dementia, including Alzheimer's disease, even though it is predominantly linked to vascular pathology. The use of tracers such as flutemetamol or florbetapir in PET scans for amyloid imaging helps identify the presence of amyloid plaques, which are a characteristic feature of Alzheimer's disease. Mixed dementia refers to the combination of vascular and Alzheimer's disease, which affects the course of therapy and clinical presentation.

For a comprehensive knowledge of the neuroanatomical and functional foundations of vascular dementia, it is imperative to integrate data from structural and functional neuroimaging. The combination of these imaging modalities leads to a more precise diagnosis, which in turn directs the development of treatment plans and other measures.

Blood Tests and Biomarkers

- **Vascular Risk Factor Assessment:**

When assessing vascular risk factors that contribute to the onset and progression of vascular dementia, blood tests are essential. Assessing lipid profiles, such as triglyceride and cholesterol levels, helps determine how atherosclerosis affects cerebral blood arteries. Hematological markers like hemoglobin A1c (HbA1c), which are particularly important for those with diabetes, offer information on long-term glycemic management.

Evaluation of inflammatory markers—like homocysteine and C-reactive protein (CRP)—is crucial because of their link to vascular disease. The risk of cerebrovascular events is increased by endothelial dysfunction and atherosclerosis, which are caused by chronic inflammation and excessive homocysteine levels.

- **Biomarkers for Neurodegeneration:**

The goal of current research on biomarkers for neurodegeneration is to find indicators that uniquely represent neuronal damage and degeneration. Neurofilament light chain (NfL) and tau protein are becoming known as possible biomarkers linked to neurodegenerative processes in vascular dementia. Increased concentrations of these biomarkers in blood or cerebrospinal fluid (CSF) might be a sign of persistent neuronal deterioration.

Blood-based biomarkers show potential for widespread clinical usage in the future since they are less intrusive than CSF biomarkers. To enable prompt intervention and individualized treatment strategies, the search for trustworthy neurodegenerative biomarkers is in line with the larger objective of early and accurate diagnosis.

- **Genetic Markers:**

The whole diagnostic assessment is influenced by genetic markers linked to vascular risk factors and vulnerability to cerebrovascular disorders. Genetic testing may be explored in patients with a strong family history or particular genetic variants linked to vascular risk factors, even though it is not a common procedure for diagnosing vascular dementia.

Comprehending the genetic terrain offers significant perspectives on a person's susceptibility to vascular disease, facilitating risk assessment and prophylactic actions. An increasingly individualized approach to the treatment of vascular dementia is made possible by the incorporation of genetic data into the diagnostic framework.

TREATMENT MODALITIES

As we go more into the field of Vascular Dementia Therapy and Management, it is important to note that the multidimensional nature of this disorder calls for a treatment strategy that incorporates several facets. Within the scope of this chapter, we investigate the various approaches that are utilized in the management of vascular dementia. These approaches range from pharmacological interventions that are aimed at addressing cognitive symptoms to non-pharmacological approaches that are designed to improve overall well-being and quality of life.

Pharmacological Interventions

- **Cholinesterase Inhibitors:**

A family of drugs called cholinesterase inhibitors, which are frequently used for Alzheimer's disease, has demonstrated some effectiveness in treating vascular dementia. The mechanism of action of these medications, which include galantamine, rivastigmine, and donepezil, is to prevent the breakdown of acetylcholine, a neurotransmitter essential to cognitive function.

Cholinesterase inhibitors are mostly used to treat cognitive loss associated with Alzheimer's disease, but they may also help people with vascular dementia. The same neurochemical abnormalities seen in both illnesses justify. These medications try to improve cholinergic neurotransmission to treat cognitive symptoms such as executive dysfunction, memory loss, and attention problems.

It's crucial to remember that each person with vascular dementia may react differently to cholinesterase inhibitors. The success of these drugs may depend on the level of neurodegeneration and vascular pathology. Notwithstanding the possible advantages, their usage needs to be carefully evaluated, taking into consideration the unique needs of each patient as well as any possible negative effects.

Memantine:

Memantine is an additional pharmaceutical treatment for vascular dementia. It is an N-methyl-D-aspartate (NMDA) receptor antagonist. Although memantine was first licensed for the treatment of Alzheimer's disease, its modes of action also point to possible advantages in vascular dementia.

Neuronal damage is linked to a process called glutamate-mediated excitotoxicity, which is facilitated by NMDA receptors. Memontine works to shield neurons from overstimulating glutamatergic activity. Given that ischemia events can initiate excitotoxic processes in cerebrovascular disorders, this neuroprotective effect is especially pertinent in this setting.

Memantine has been used in vascular dementia clinical studies, where it has been shown to enhance cognitive function and activities of daily living. Depending on the clinical presentation and patient reaction, the medication may be included in the treatment plan either alone or in conjunction with cholinesterase inhibitors.

- **Emerging Therapies:**

The field of pharmacological therapies for vascular dementia is constantly evolving, with new therapeutic approaches being the subject of continuous study. As our understanding of the intricate pathophysiology behind vascular dementia continues to develop, several drugs targeting neuroinflammation, oxidative stress, and vascular health are being investigated.

Medication that directly addresses risk factors for cardiovascular disease is one promising field of research. By addressing the underlying vascular pathology, antihypertensive medications, statins, and antiplatelet medications, for instance, may be able to prevent or delay the onset of vascular dementia. Clinical trials are investigating how these drugs affect cognitive function and the course of the disease.

Moreover, the goal of studying growth-promoting compounds and neurotrophic factors is to promote the regeneration and repair of neurons. These new treatments have the potential to change the course of vascular dementia by treating its underlying causes as well as its symptoms.

Non-pharmacological Approaches

- **Cognitive Rehabilitation:**

For those with vascular dementia, cognitive rehabilitation is a non-pharmacological strategy that aims to enhance daily living abilities and cognitive function. The objective is to extend the person's independence and improve their capacity to carry out daily tasks.

Programs for cognitive rehabilitation are customized to each person's unique cognitive deficiencies. They frequently include organized drills and activities aimed at improving executive function, memory, focus, and problem-solving skills. Therapists collaborate closely with patients and others who are caring for them to create coping mechanisms and adjustments for cognitive function impairments.

Research shows that cognitive rehabilitation can lead to gains in cognitive performance and functional capacities in patients with vascular dementia. It offers a customized, all-encompassing method of addressing the disease's cognitive effects, encouraging confidence and a sense of success in day-to-day tasks.

- **Physical Exercise:**

One effective non-pharmacological technique for the treatment of vascular dementia is physical activity. Frequent exercise has been linked to several cognitive advantages, such as enhanced executive, memory, and attention spans. Exercise also helps to control vascular risk factors in the context of vascular dementia.

Walking, swimming, and cycling are examples of aerobic activities that have been found to improve cognitive performance. Exercise increases neuroplasticity, stimulates blood flow to the brain, and may even aid in the development of new neurons. It also aids in treating diseases like diabetes and hypertension, lowering the risk of stroke, and preserving cardiovascular health.

Strength training and balance exercises are also key components of an exercise program for patients with vascular dementia. These exercises improve physical health in general and lower the chance of falls, which can be especially harmful to those who suffer from cognitive impairment.

- **Music and Art Therapy:**

Innovative non-pharmacological techniques that engage the creative and emotional sides of people suffering from vascular dementia include music therapy and art therapy. These treatments acknowledge the power of music and art to arouse emotions, bring back memories, and provide persons who might find it difficult to communicate verbally a way to express themselves.

A person receiving music therapy may choose to sing, play an instrument, or listen to music that suits their tastes and talents. Research has demonstrated that music therapy can help people with vascular dementia feel better emotionally, behave less agitatedly, and think more clearly. It can pique people's emotions deeply, resulting in happy moments and bonds.

Drawing, painting, and sculpting are just a few of the visual arts activities that are included in art therapy. The act of creating may be therapeutic, giving people a way to communicate and express themselves. In patients with vascular dementia, art therapy has been linked to improvements in mood, cognitive function, and general well-being.

These non-pharmacological methods provide a person-centered and comprehensive approach to treatment by acknowledging the uniqueness of every person with vascular dementia. They provide opportunities for emotional expression, meaningful interaction, and cognitive stimulation, all of which enhance quality of life.

CAREGIVER SUPPORT

It becomes clear as we traverse the complex terrain of vascular dementia therapy and management that caregiver support is a crucial part of receiving all-encompassing treatment. People who are caring for someone with vascular dementia frequently need help and understanding from their carers, who are essential in handling the practical parts of care as well as offering emotional support and preserving their wellbeing. This chapter examines the value of respite care alternatives, methods for offering emotional support, and caregiver engagement in the setting of vascular dementia.

Importance of Caregiver Involvement

- **The Complexities of Vascular Dementia Care:**

Because vascular dementia has certain features, caring for someone with the condition can be difficult and demanding. Vascular dementia frequently has behavioral and psychological symptoms that might differ greatly from person to person along with cognitive impairment. Aggression, anger, mood swings, and communication issues are a few of these signs.

Caregiving is further complicated by the unpredictable nature of vascular dementia, which progresses gradually and can cause abrupt cognitive impairments following vascular incidents. Caregivers need to overcome these obstacles while continuing to take a patient and caring stance.

- **Involvement in Daily Activities:**

Involving caregivers in the everyday routines of patients with vascular dementia is essential. Falling cognitive function can make it difficult for people to do things like take a shower, dress, and take their prescriptions. To supply the required assistance, encourage independence when it is feasible, and adjust to the individual's changing requirements, caregivers are essential.

Together, participating in activities like hobbies, walks, or cognitive exercises improves the relationship between the caregiver and the person suffering from vascular dementia while also enhancing the individual's quality of life. Keeping a regular daily schedule helps reduce uncertainty and anxiety and provides the person receiving care and themselves a sense of security.

- **Monitoring and Managing Health:**

Diabetes and cardiovascular problems are two prevalent medical disorders that frequently combine with vascular dementia. In addition to making sure that prescriptions are taken as directed and arranging for routine check-ups with medical specialists, caregivers are essential in the monitoring and management of various coexisting health issues.

Caregivers must also be alert for any indications of acute health problems, such as infections or cardiovascular events, which can seriously impair the mental and physical health of patients suffering from vascular dementia. One of the most important aspects of caregiver involvement is having the ability to effectively communicate with healthcare providers and speak up for the needs of the individual.

Providing Emotional Support

- **Understanding the Emotional Impact:**

It is emotionally taxing to care for a person with vascular dementia, and caregivers may feel a range of emotions as they see their loved one's cognitive abilities deteriorate, including despair, anger, guilt, and even bereavement. Providing effective emotional support begins with understanding and accepting these emotions.

Because vascular dementia progresses, caregivers may experience both ongoing caregiving and mourning for the person they once knew. It might be helpful for caregivers to acknowledge the legitimacy of these emotions and seek support via professional help, organizations, or therapy.

- **Communication Strategies:**

The foundation of emotional support in dementia care is effective communication. People suffering from vascular dementia may find it difficult to express themselves verbally as their cognitive abilities deteriorate, which can cause irritation and even communication breakdowns. To improve comprehension and lessen stress, caregivers can use a variety of communication techniques.

- Make your wording plain and uncomplicated.
- Divide instructions and tasks into digestible steps.

- Give the person some time to answer, and exercise patience.
- To communicate meaning, use nonverbal clues like gestures and facial expressions.
- Take note of the person's emotions and body language.

- **Creating a Supportive Environment:**

For those suffering from vascular dementia, their emotional state can be greatly impacted by their physical surroundings. Caregivers can provide a comforting and encouraging atmosphere by:

- Reducing confusion by clearing out clutter and making clear paths.

- Ensuring adequate illumination to improve vision.

- Including cherished trinkets like family pictures, or other familiar and reassuring stuff.

- Establishing regular times and being consistent with everyday tasks.

- **Respecting Individuality:**

Sustaining a sense of self and uniqueness is essential for the mental health of those suffering from vascular dementia. To help with this, caregivers can:

- Encouraging pursuits that fit the individual's interests and inclinations.

- Honoring individual preferences, whether they relate to daily schedules or attire.
- Honoring successes and happy times, no matter how tiny.

The process of offering emotional support is dynamic and continuous, and it changes as the illness worsens. Caregivers greatly enhance the emotional well-being of both themselves and the people they look after by recognizing the emotional impact, using good communication techniques, fostering a supportive atmosphere, and appreciating uniqueness.

Respite Care Options

- **The Need for Respite:**

Providing care for an individual suffering from vascular dementia is an arduous and unrelenting obligation that may have an adverse effect on the mental and physical health of the caregiver. Periodic breaks sometimes referred to as respite care, are essential to avoiding burnout, preserving the health of caregivers, and maintaining the standard of care given to the patient with vascular dementia.

With the help of short-term respite, caregivers may take a break from their caregiving duties and rejuvenate. It can come in several forms, such as adult day programs, in-home respite care, and short-term residential care alternatives.

- **In-Home Respite Care:**

In-home respite care is sending volunteers or qualified experts into the house to take care of the person with vascular dementia while the primary caregiver takes a break. There are several advantages to this type of respite care:

- Comfortable and Known Environment: By keeping the person in a known setting, regular disturbances are less likely.
- Personalized Care: Care may be customized to meet each person's unique requirements and preferences.

- Temporary Relief: During this time, caregivers can rest, take care of themselves, or attend to personal needs.

In-home respite care offers caregivers the freedom to refuel while maintaining the safety of their loved ones. It may include companionship, monitoring, and help with everyday tasks.

- **Adult Day Programs:**

Adult day programs provide supervised, organized activities in a group environment for people with dementia. These programs allow caregivers to sign up their loved ones for a part of the day, giving them a vacation from their caring duties. Adult day programs include several benefits.

- Social Engagement: Taking part in worthwhile activities and interacting socially with peers is beneficial to participants.
- Professional Supervision: Skilled employees supervise the operations and offer support as needed.
- Cognitive Stimulation: Engaging in activities aimed at enhancing cognitive function improves participants' general well-being.

While their loved ones are enrolled in adult day programs, caregivers can utilize that time to concentrate on personal projects, take care of themselves, or just relax.

- **Short-Term Residential Care:**

Caregivers can take longer breaks from their caregiving duties when they choose short-term residential care choices like assisted living communities or respite care centers. This type of care is especially helpful when caregivers require longer periods away from their duties, such as when they go on vacation or have personal obligations.

People with vascular dementia who are receiving short-term residential care are provided with complete care in a professional environment. With this option, caregivers can take care of their own health needs, take care of family concerns, or just take a vacation from the daily rigors of caring.

In addition to being vital for the health of carers, respite care raises the standard of care given to patients with vascular dementia. Caregivers can maintain their capacity to deliver effective and compassionate care for an extended period by implementing respite care alternatives into their caregiving strategy.

LIFESTYLE MODIFICATIONS

Alterations to one's way of life, which can have a beneficial effect on one's cognitive performance and general well-being, are included in the holistic approach to the treatment and management of vascular dementia. This approach goes beyond the use of medicinal therapies. This chapter examines important aspects of lifestyle, such as diet and nutrition, cognitive stimulation, and the control of cardiovascular risk factors. It provides insights into how these alterations might help the holistic care of persons who have vascular dementia.

Diet and Nutrition

- ## The Impact of Diet on Vascular Health:

Adopting a heart-healthy diet can help manage vascular dementia, as nutrition plays a critical role in vascular health. Essential nutrients can be obtained while limiting the consumption of trans and saturated fats by eating a diet high in fruits, vegetables, whole grains, and lean meats.

Particularly the Mediterranean diet has drawn interest due to its possible advantages in maintaining cognitive function. This diet places special emphasis on:

- Fruits and vegetables: Packed with vitamins and antioxidants that promote good health overall, including mental wellness.
- Omega-3 fatty acids, which are abundant in fish, have been linked to a lower incidence of cognitive impairment.
- An excellent source of monounsaturated fats that may protect the brain is olive oil.
- Nuts and seeds: supply antioxidants, other nutrients, and good fats.

- **Hydration and Cognitive Function:**

It's critical to be well hydrated for general health, as dehydration can negatively affect cognitive performance. Dehydration can occur in people with vascular dementia for a variety of reasons, including forgetfulness, problems identifying thirst, or difficulties controlling fluid consumption on their own.

People with vascular dementia should have their water levels monitored and encouraged by caregivers and healthcare professionals. Water-rich meal offerings, regular fluid intake intervals, and easy access to liquids all day long are some strategies. Sustaining the ideal level of water promotes general health and cognitive performance.

- **Nutritional Supplements:**

All the nutrients that are required should ideally be found in a well-balanced diet, however, some people with vascular dementia may benefit from taking supplements. Certain nutrients have been linked to improved cognitive function, including vitamin D, omega-3 fatty acids, and vitamin B complex.

But it's important to use caution while supplementing and get medical advice from qualified doctors. Everybody has different nutritional needs, and taking too many supplements might be harmful. The emphasis should always be on getting nutrients from a varied, nutrient-rich diet.

Cognitive Stimulation

- **The Importance of Cognitive Engagement:**

For those suffering from vascular dementia, cognitive stimulation is an essential part of changing their lifestyle. Mentally demanding activities can strengthen brain connections, support cognitive function, and possibly even halt the advancement of cognitive decline.

Cognitive stimulation comes from mentally taxing activities like reading, playing games, solving puzzles, and picking up new abilities. To keep these activities fun and attainable, caregivers and medical experts should adapt them to the person's skills and preferences.

- **Cognitive Rehabilitation Programs:**

People with vascular dementia can benefit from focused cognitive exercises provided by structured cognitive rehabilitation programs run by qualified specialists. To boost cognitive capacities and improve day-to-day functioning, these programs concentrate on certain cognitive domains, such as memory, attention, and executive function.

Personalized goal-setting, ongoing evaluations, and modification of therapies in response to the patient's development are all part of cognitive rehabilitation. Cognitive rehabilitation may not be able to change the underlying vascular illness, but it can help to maximize the quality of life and cognitive function.

- **Social Engagement:**

A potent kind of cognitive stimulation that improves general well-being is social involvement. People with vascular dementia can participate in cognitive tasks by maintaining social connections, taking part in group activities, and cultivating meaningful relationships.

Whether via participation in group activities created especially for people with dementia, family get-togethers, or community events, caregivers and healthcare professionals should support and encourage social contacts. Beyond just improving cognitive function, social involvement also improves emotional health and lessens feelings of loneliness.

Managing Cardiovascular Risk Factors

- **Hypertension Management:**

Vascular dementia is closely linked to hypertension, or high blood pressure, as a major cardiovascular risk factor. Maintaining a healthy blood pressure range is essential to stop more brain vascular injury. Among the lifestyle changes that can help control blood pressure are:

- Changing to a low-sodium diet: Cutting less on salt can help control blood pressure.
- Regular physical activity: Exercise helps to maintain blood pressure and cardiovascular health.

- Taking antihypertensive drugs as directed: Maintaining hypertension management requires adherence to the recommended drug schedule.

The management of hypertension in patients with vascular dementia necessitates regular blood pressure monitoring and close coordination with healthcare professionals.

- **Diabetes Control:**

Type 2 diabetes in particular is a cardiovascular risk factor that might exacerbate cognitive deterioration. For those with diabetes and vascular dementia, controlling blood glucose levels through lifestyle changes is essential. Important tactics consist of:

- Following a low-glycemic, balanced diet: limiting additional sugars, selecting lean meats, and complete grains.
- Regularly partaking in physical activity: Cardiovascular health and glycemic management are enhanced by exercise.
- Using antidiabetic prescription drugs: Medication adherence is necessary to keep blood sugar under control.

To ensure effective diabetes treatment, there has to be careful collaboration between healthcare practitioners, people with vascular dementia, and those who are caring for them.

- **Cholesterol and Lipid Management:**

A higher risk of atherosclerosis and vascular events is linked to elevated cholesterol levels, especially low-density lipoprotein (LDL) cholesterol. Lifestyle changes can help with lipid management:

- Eating a diet low in cholesterol: putting a focus on nutritious grains, fruits, veggies, and healthy fat sources.
- Physical exercise regularly: Exercise improves cholesterol levels.
- Taking cholesterol-lowering drugs as directed: When dietary changes alone aren't enough to control cholesterol levels, doctors may recommend medication.

- To optimize cholesterol management and lower cardiovascular risk, regular lipid monitoring and cooperation with healthcare specialists are crucial.

LEGAL AND ETHICAL CONSIDERATIONS

It is not enough to just implement lifestyle and medical therapies to successfully navigate the complexity of vascular dementia; one must also pay special attention to the ethical and legal aspects involved. When it comes to the care of people who have vascular dementia, this chapter delves into important topics such as advance care planning, guardianship, power of attorney, and ethical concerns that may emerge.

Advance Care Planning

- **Understanding Advance Care Planning:**

For people with vascular dementia, advance care planning is an essential part of moral and patient-centered treatment. In this process, desires for future healthcare are discussed, particularly in light of probable cognitive impairment, with patients, their families, and healthcare professionals.

Important components of advance care planning consist of:

- A living will is a written statement of a person's choices for life-sustaining procedures and medical interventions if they are unable to communicate or make their own decisions.

- Healthcare Proxy or Surrogate Decision Maker: Designating a reliable individual to handle healthcare choices if the principal is incapacitated.

- **Timing and Sensitivity in Discussions:**

It takes tact and compassion to bring up advanced care planning when speaking with someone whose cognitive and emotional states are impaired. It is best to start these conversations early in the course of the illness so that the person affected may communicate their desires while still capable of doing so.

Healthcare professionals and caregivers should approach these conversations empathetically and deliver information that is easy to grasp. Advance care plans must be reviewed and updated if the patient's choices change and the condition develops.

- **Documenting and Sharing Preferences:**

Once preferences have been determined, they have to be recorded in legally enforceable papers such as healthcare proxy forms and living wills. Healthcare professionals, family members, and other caregivers for patients with vascular dementia must have easy access to these records.

By registering preferences, people may make sure that their beliefs and desires are respected while making healthcare decisions. By providing this information to caregivers and the medical staff, disputes are reduced and continuity of treatment is encouraged.

Guardianship and Power of Attorney

- **Guardianship:**

People with vascular dementia may eventually become unable to make wise judgments regarding their financial and personal matters as the condition worsens. In certain situations, guardianship could be required. A court-appointed guardian is designated to make decisions on behalf of the person who is considered incapacitated through the procedure of guardianship.

Guardianship is a big decision that might affect someone's autonomy, thus it should only be taken after carefully weighing the person's best interests. Financial, residential, and healthcare decisions may be made by the designated guardian.

- **Power of Attorney:**

A Power of Attorney (POA) is a legal instrument that gives someone the right to act as another person's agent and make decisions. It enables people to name a reliable representative to handle financial, legal, and occasionally medical decisions on their behalf.

There are several kinds of POAs, such as:

- A general power of attorney gives the named individual extensive decision-making authority.

- Durable Power of Attorney: Continues to function in the event of the principal's incapacitation.
- Healthcare Power of Attorney: Deals specifically with choices about medical treatment and care.

Establishing a power of attorney requires selecting a dependable and trustworthy person. The paper must be understandable, legitimate legally, and compliant with the relevant local legislation.

- **Balancing Autonomy and Protection:**

Making decisions about guardianship and power of attorney requires striking a careful balance between preserving the person's autonomy and making sure they are taken care of. It is important to include individuals suffering from vascular dementia as much as possible in these decision-making processes, keeping their desires and preferences in mind.

To safeguard the interests of the person, the least restrictive measures should be given priority in the process. It is imperative to conduct frequent evaluations of an individual's competence and to periodically evaluate guardianship and power of attorney arrangements to guarantee that decisions are in line with the person's changing demands and ideals.

Ethical Issues in Vascular Dementia Care

- **Person-Centered Care and Autonomy:**

The concepts of person-centered care and respect for autonomy are fundamental to the ethical issues in the treatment of vascular dementia. Vascular dementia causes cognitive deterioration, which can be problematic, but it is important to acknowledge and respect the humanity of those who have the disease.

Person-centered care entails adjusting the level of treatment to each patient's preferences, capabilities, and values. This method calls for maintaining constant contact, allowing the person with vascular dementia to participate in decision-making to the greatest degree feasible, and honoring their right to autonomy.

- **Informed Consent and Shared Decision-Making:**

A fundamental component of moral medical practice is informed consent. However, people with vascular dementia may find it difficult to give their informed permission for medical procedures when their cognitive impairment worsens. In these situations, collaborative decision-making including dementia patients, their relatives, and medical professionals becomes essential.

Healthcare providers have to make an effort to prioritize interventions that are in line with the patient's values and quality of life, including family members or caregivers in conversations, and provide information in a way that the patient can understand.

- **End-of-Life Decision-Making:**

Complex ethical issues are raised by end-of-life decisions in the care of patients with vascular dementia. Decisions on artificial feeding and hydration, the use of life-sustaining therapies, and the general objectives of care may need to be made by patients, caregivers, and healthcare professionals.

The concepts of beneficence respecting the person's comfort and dignity and non-maleficence avoidance of needless suffering—should serve as guidance for these choices. To guarantee that choices for end-of-life care are in line with the patient's beliefs and desires, ethical talks concerning this matter should include the vascular dementia patient, their healthcare staff, and family members.

- **Dignity and Quality of Life:**

Basic ethical requirements include upholding the dignity of people suffering from vascular dementia and placing a high value on their quality of life. This entails attending to psychological and emotional demands in addition to physiological ones.

It is the goal of caregivers and healthcare professionals to provide surroundings that uphold privacy, support dignity, and facilitate meaningful interaction. Methods like music therapy, person-centered activities, and memory therapy improve the general dignity and well-being of people with vascular dementia.

- **Ethical Considerations in Research:**

Vascular dementia research presents ethical questions about participant autonomy, informed consent, and the possible advantages and disadvantages of therapies. Extra precautions must be taken to protect participants' rights and welfare in research involving people with cognitive impairments.

A thorough ethical examination of research methods is necessary to guarantee that involvement is voluntary, that consent is obtained where feasible from people with cognitive impairment, and that risks are kept to a minimum. Research ethics preserve the values of beneficence and respect for human beings while promoting scientific advancement.

RESEARCH AND FUTURE DIRECTIONS

Constant research attempts have a vital role in creating the landscape of diagnosis, treatment, and management of vascular dementia. This is because our understanding of vascular dementia is always evolving. The present status of research, ongoing clinical trials, interesting areas of inquiry, and prospective breakthroughs in the field of vascular dementia are all discussed in depth in this chapter.

Ongoing Clinical Trials

- **Advancements in Therapeutic Interventions:**

A vital method for evaluating the security and effectiveness of cutting-edge treatment approaches for vascular dementia is clinical trials. Extant clinical studies investigate various methodologies, such as pharmacological medicines that target certain pathways linked to vascular disease, lifestyle interventions, and combination therapy.

One prominent field of research is medications that directly target risk factors for cardiovascular disease. Not only are antihypertensive drugs, statins, and antiplatelet medicines being studied for their

97

effects on cardiovascular health but also for their potential to affect how vascular dementia develops. The purpose of these trials is to determine whether treating diseases like hypertension and hyperlipidemia will slow down cognitive aging and enhance overall results.

Furthermore, neuroprotective drugs that might mitigate the effects of cerebrovascular accidents are gaining popularity. Antioxidants, anti-inflammatory medicines, and pharmaceuticals that target neurodegenerative pathways are a few examples of these compounds. The purpose of ongoing trials is to evaluate these substances' effectiveness and safety in people with vascular dementia.

- **Cognitive Rehabilitation and Non-Pharmacological Approaches:**

The efficacy of non-pharmacological therapies and cognitive rehabilitation in treating vascular dementia is also being investigated in clinical studies. These interventions include physical activity regimens, structured cognitive exercises, and psychosocial therapies targeted at enhancing mood, cognitive performance, and general quality of life.

Trials of cognitive rehabilitation frequently entail individualized treatments designed to address each person's unique cognitive impairments. To optimize the impact of these treatments, researchers are examining the best timing, level of intensity, and length of time to implement them. Furthermore, non-pharmacological methods including art therapy, music therapy, and sensory stimulation are being investigated for their ability to improve cognitive performance and overall well-being in patients with vascular dementia.

- **Biomarkers for Early Diagnosis and Monitoring:**

Novel approaches to the identification of biomarkers linked to vascular dementia have been made possible by developments in neuroimaging and molecular biology. Validating and improving these indicators to allow for earlier diagnosis and more precise tracking of illness development is the main goal of ongoing clinical research.

Researchers can see both anatomical and functional changes in the brain thanks to neuroimaging techniques like positron emission tomography (PET) and magnetic resonance imaging (MRI). The diagnostic and prognostic use of vascular pathology-related biomarkers, such as cerebral microbleeds, white matter hyperintensities, and changes in cerebral blood flow, is being studied.

Additionally being studied are blood-based biomarkers, such as certain proteins and genetic markers. These biomarkers may be useful for identifying patients at risk and tracking the course of the disease. They may also provide light on the underlying pathophysiology of vascular dementia.

Promising Areas of Research

- **Vascular Health and Cognitive Aging:**

Studies examining the complex connection between vascular health and cognitive aging have become more well-known. Research is being conducted to determine how vascular risk factors—such as diabetes, hypertension, and hyperlipidemia—affect cognitive aging across time. Developing focused therapies and preventative measures requires an understanding of the vascular contributions to dementia and cognitive impairment (VCID).

Research on the effects of pharmaceutical therapies, vascular risk factor management, and lifestyle changes on cognitive outcomes appears promising. To enable therapies that target both vascular and neurodegenerative elements of the illness, researchers are working to understand the intricate interactions between these processes.

- **Precision Medicine Approaches:**

Precision medicine is making great strides toward customizing therapies to the specific needs of patients with vascular dementia. Variations in lifestyle, genetics, and the existence of certain vascular risk factors can all impact how the condition develops. The potential of a precision medicine strategy to tailor treatment plans to specific patient profiles is still being investigated.

The goal of genomic research is to find genetic markers linked to a higher risk of vascular dementia. Comprehending the genetic foundations of the illness might pave the way for focused treatments and customized approaches. To generate complete and customized treatment regimens, precision medicine techniques also take lifestyle variables, pharmaceutical reactions, and comorbidities into account.

- **Multimodal Interventions:**

The potential advantages of multimodal interventions—which target many elements of vascular dementia simultaneously—are being investigated more and more in research. To build complete and synergistic methods, these therapies may incorporate lifestyle adjustments, cognitive rehabilitation, pharmaceutical treatments, and control of vascular risk factors.

Multimodal therapies acknowledge the complexity of vascular dementia and the possibility that different components of the illness may not be adequately addressed by a single strategy. The goal of ongoing research is to clarify the best combinations of therapies when to use them, and how they work together to improve cognitive results.

Potential Breakthroughs

- **Disease-Modifying Therapies:**

The hunt for treatments that alter the condition is a fundamental aspect of vascular dementia research. There is an urgent need for therapies that can change the course of the illness, reducing or stopping its advancement, even though the majority of present medications concentrate on managing symptoms.

A new study investigates drugs that target certain pathways related to neurodegeneration, neuroinflammation, and vascular disease. These promising developments seek to treat the underlying processes of vascular dementia in addition to improving cognitive symptoms.

107

The potential of clinical trials examining disease-modifying medicines to alter the therapy landscape is closely observed.

- **Artificial Intelligence and Predictive Modeling:**

In the realm of vascular dementia research, artificial intelligence (AI) and machine learning have become highly effective instruments. These technologies are promising for the prediction of cognitive decline, the identification of those who are more likely to acquire vascular dementia, and the improvement of treatment plans.

AI-powered predictive modeling examines enormous datasets, including genetic, clinical, and neuroimaging data. AI has the potential to aid in the early detection of high-risk patients through the discovery of patterns and correlations, hence facilitating prompt interventions and customized treatment regimens. The potential of AI to transform risk prediction and prognostic modeling in vascular dementia is being investigated in this field through ongoing research.

- **Vascular Cognitive Impairment Subtypes:**

According to a recent study, vascular cognitive impairment might not be a single, homogenous condition but rather a continuum with several subgroups. Determining and describing these subgroups might be a significant discovery that results in more specialized and customized treatments.

When subtyping vascular cognitive impairment, variables including the pattern of cognitive impairments, the location of vascular lesions, and the existence of certain risk factors are taken into account. Treatment choices may be influenced by knowledge of the variability within vascular dementia, enabling more individualized and successful therapies based on each patient's unique clinical profile.

GLOBAL PERSPECTIVES ON VASCULAR DEMENTIA

The signs and symptoms of vascular dementia are experienced all over the world, and how it is diagnosed, treated, and cared for differs greatly from one culture and location to another. This chapter examines the various perspectives on vascular dementia that are held around the world. It highlights the differences in diagnosis and treatment approaches, as well as the cultural factors that play a role in determining the care that is provided to individuals who have this complicated condition.

Variances in Diagnosis and Treatment Approaches

- **Regional Differences in Diagnosis:**

Numerous factors, such as the availability of diagnostic resources, the healthcare system, and the frequency of vascular risk factors, affect the diagnosis of vascular dementia. People may have greater access to sophisticated neuroimaging methods, cognitive evaluations, and specialized dementia clinics in high-income nations with developed healthcare systems, enabling more precise and prompt diagnosis.

On the other hand, healthcare inequities and few resources may provide difficulties for low- and middle-income nations. In these circumstances, the diagnosis of vascular dementia could depend more on clinical judgments, and neuroimaging resources might not be as easily accessible. This may lead to an underdiagnosis or delayed diagnosis, which will affect when the right assistance and treatments are started.

- **Treatment Disparities and Access to Care:**

Global disparities in the management of vascular dementia are a result of differences in the accessibility of specialist care and the availability of therapeutic choices. People with vascular dementia may be able to access a variety of pharmaceutical and non-pharmacological therapies, such as cognitive-enhancing drugs, rehabilitative programs, and multidisciplinary care teams, in areas with strong healthcare systems.

On the other hand, access to these therapies can be restricted in environments with few resources. Treatment discrepancies may also be influenced by variables including the cost of medications, the accessibility of medical personnel with dementia care training, and public perceptions of cognitive health. An interdisciplinary strategy that includes legislative modifications, educational programs, and infrastructural improvements in the healthcare system is needed to address these inequities.

- **Challenges in Multinational Research:**

International views on vascular dementia are influenced by difficulties in undertaking multidisciplinary research as well as geographical differences in healthcare. Obstacles in clinical trials and research are frequently associated with heterogeneous patient populations, disparities in regulations, and discrepancies in healthcare systems.

To improve our knowledge of vascular dementia and provide treatments that work for a range of patients, coordination of research endeavors and international collaboration are crucial. In the end, multinational research projects can contribute to more broadly applicable recommendations for diagnosis and treatment by assisting in the identification of common patterns, risk factors, and successful therapies.

Cultural Considerations in Care

- **Stigma and Cultural Attitudes:**

The experiences of people with dementia and those who care for them are greatly influenced by cultural views on dementia, particularly vascular dementia. The stigma attached to cognitive decline can differ greatly throughout cultures, which has an impact on people's and families' willingness to ask for assistance and reveal symptoms.

Certain cultural groups may be reluctant to talk about or admit cognitive deficits because they are afraid of the affected person being socially isolated or because they are worried about how the community will see them. To combat cultural stigma, it is necessary to implement culturally aware education and awareness initiatives that encourage early detection and support service access.

- **Family Dynamics and Caregiving:**

Cultural differences in family structures and traditions around caregiving have an impact on how people with vascular dementia are cared for. There may be a strong cultural history of family caregivers, in which family members assume the main responsibility for providing care for their ailing loved ones. In certain cases, there may be a greater emphasis on formal care services.

To effectively assist family dynamics, one must comprehend and honor cultural differences. Healthcare practitioners need to interact with families in a manner that conforms to cultural norms, recognizing the significance of extended family members and taking into account the influence of cultural norms on caregiving obligations.

- **Language and Communication Challenges:**

Culturally competent treatment for patients with vascular dementia might be significantly hampered by communication difficulties and language obstacles. Healthcare workers must use techniques that guarantee efficient communication in multicultural communities or when patients and caregivers have different language origins.

Understanding cultural quirks in communication methods, preferences, and expectations is just as important to cultural competency in healthcare as language proficiency. To ensure that people and their families receive thorough and understandable information regarding vascular dementia and its care, individuals must have access to interpreters and culturally appropriate communication tools to overcome language gaps.

- **Traditional Healing Practices and Complementary Therapies:**

Cultural viewpoints on health frequently include complementary and alternative therapies in addition to regular medical treatments. In certain societies, people could consult traditional healers or use herbal treatments in their medical routine.

Healthcare providers need to be open and respectful of these cultural customs and acknowledge that they could coexist with medical interventions. Care plans that are comprehensive and culturally appropriate may be developed by having cooperative conversations with patients and their families on the integration of conventional practices with evidence-based medicine.

CASE STUDIES

Real-life case studies offer useful insights into the many symptoms, treatment options, and problems connected with vascular dementia. Vascular dementia offers a clinical landscape that is complicated and nuanced, and these case studies give valuable insights. In this chapter, we investigate real-life instances of vascular dementia cases, look into the results of therapy, and talk about the difficulties that are experienced when treating people who have this complex neurocognitive illness.

Real-life Examples of Vascular Dementia Cases

- **Case Study 1: Mr. A - The Silent Strokes**

Mr. Anthony, a 72-year-old man with a history of diabetes and hypertension, showed here with mild cognitive impairments that his family recognized. He had a deterioration in executive functions, had trouble recalling recent events, and became lost in familiar environments. A succession of quiet strokes and tiny ischemia lesions in different brain areas were discovered by neuroimaging.

This example demonstrates the subtle character of vascular dementia, a condition in which a series of little strokes gradually impair cognitive function. There were no obvious neurological signs, but there was a noticeable effect on cognitive performance. In many situations, the difficulty is in identifying the problem early and taking action to stop the cognitive decline from getting worse.

- **Case Study 2: Mrs. B - The Vascular Cognitive Impairment**

Mrs. Benitra, a 65-year-old lady, came in with a history of growing memory loss and repeated transient ischemic attacks (TIAs). Neuropsychological evaluations revealed deficits in executive function, memory, and attention. Significant white matter hyperintensities and signs of chronic cerebral hypoperfusion were found by imaging tests.

This example illustrates the range of cognitive impairment caused by vascular dysfunction, wherein cognitive abnormalities are identified. Addressing the underlying vascular risk factors, maximizing cerebral perfusion, and offering specialized cognitive therapies to enhance everyday functioning are the key challenges in managing such instances.

- **Case Study 3: Mr. C - Mixed Etiology Dementia**

Mr. Carl, an 80-year-old man, had a complicated clinical picture that included vascular pathology and Alzheimer's disease. He showed signs of deteriorating memory, trouble speaking and thinking clearly, and poor judgment. Vascular lesions and the brain atrophy typical of Alzheimer's disease were both detected by neuroimaging.

The difficulty in differentiating between dementia with a single vascular cause and dementia with a mixed etiology, in which several disease processes contribute to cognitive deterioration, is brought to light by this example. Precise diagnosis and treatment planning depends on thorough evaluations, such as biomarker research and neuroimaging.

Treatment Outcomes and Challenges

- **Pharmacological Interventions: Cholinesterase Inhibitors and Memantine**

Pharmacological therapies for vascular dementia management are intended to reduce cognitive symptoms and enhance day-to-day functioning. It is normal practice to administer cholinesterase inhibitors, such as galantamine, rivastigmine, and donepezil, to improve cholinergic neurotransmission. Memantine is an antagonist of the N-methyl-D-aspartate (NMDA) receptor that may be used to control glutamatergic neurotransmission either by itself or in conjunction with cholinesterase inhibitors.

Individual differences exist in the outcomes of treatment; some show very slight gains in daily functioning and cognitive abilities. However reactions to medication changes can be erratic, and not everyone with vascular dementia experiences meaningful improvement. The possibility of adverse effects, variations in treatment response, and the requirement for close observation are among the difficulties.

- **Emerging Therapies and Clinical Trials**

Treatment options for vascular dementia are changing as a result of continuous research into novel treatments. Clinical trials investigate new pharmacological medicines, such as anti-inflammatory medications, antioxidants, and substances that affect illness, and target vascular and neurodegenerative pathways.

Investigations into treatment results from developing medicines continue, and difficulties persist in converting encouraging preclinical data into practical clinical interventions. Furthermore, it might be difficult to identify subgroups with vascular dementia that could react better to particular therapies due to the variety of the disease.

- **Non-pharmacological Approaches: Cognitive Rehabilitation, Physical Exercise, and Music Therapy**

A vital part of the comprehensive care of vascular dementia is the use of non-pharmacological therapies. Programs for cognitive rehabilitation use systematic exercises and techniques to improve particular cognitive domains. Engaging in physical activity, such as resistance and aerobic training, improves vascular health overall and may have a beneficial effect on cognitive performance. People are emotionally and cognitively engaged by music therapy, which opens up channels for communication and expression.

Comorbidities, dementia stage, and the patient's level of participation all frequently impact the results of nonpharmacological treatment. Difficulties include the requirement for customized and specific interventions, possible participation hurdles, and differences in treatment compliance.

- **Caregiver Support: Importance, Challenges, and Respite Care**

Involving caregivers is essential to provide patients with vascular dementia with complete care. The well-being of the person receiving care as well as that of the caregiver is influenced by possibilities for respite care, emotional support, and aid with everyday tasks. The psychological toll of seeing a loved one's cognitive decline, the physical strain of providing care, and striking a balance between the requirements of the individual and the well-being of the caregiver are all obstacles in the way of providing caregiver assistance.

To avoid caregiver burnout and maintain long-term caring efforts, respite care is crucial. Financial limitations, a lack of professional caregiving services, and the requirement for cultural competency in care delivery are some of the obstacles to obtaining respite care.

- **Ethical Considerations: Advance Care Planning and End-of-life Decision-making**

Early in the course of the disease, advance care planning conversations are crucial when it comes to vascular dementia care from an ethical standpoint. People are urged to voice their views on medical interventions, life-sustaining treatments, and designating healthcare proxies or surrogate decision-makers due to the possibility of cognitive impairment.

Advance care planning is fraught with difficulties, such as cultural differences in attitudes toward dying conversations, the impact of family dynamics on the process of making decisions, and the need to make sure that the wishes communicated are consistent with the person's changing moral principles. When making decisions concerning end-of-life care, ethical issues are taken into account. It is crucial to talk about the objectives of care, the use of life-sustaining therapies, and palliative care choices.

CONCLUSION

A complicated subtype of neurocognitive disease that combines the fields of vascular pathology and cognitive decline is vascular dementia. We have examined many aspects of vascular dementia in this thorough investigation, including its definition, prevalence, diagnosis, treatment options, caregiver assistance, ethical and legal issues, worldwide viewpoints, and real-world case studies. We review important ideas as we come to the end of our exploration of the world of vascular dementia and consider the promise that comes from continuing research and changing viewpoints.

Hope for the Future

Developments in Research and Treatment Interventions: Thanks to continuing research and improvements in therapeutic interventions, there is hope for those suffering from vascular dementia in the future. Clinical trials are a means to change the face of therapy and provide hope for more efficacious interventions by investigating novel pharmacological agents, developing therapeutics, and disease-modifying strategies.

Interventions may be tailored to individual profiles with the use of precision medicine, artificial intelligence, and a better knowledge of vascular cognitive impairment subtypes.

Developments in disease-modifying treatments may change how vascular dementia progresses by treating both the underlying processes and cognitive symptoms of the condition.

Multidisciplinary Methods and Holistic Treatment: As vascular dementia takes on more facets, multidisciplinary approaches and holistic care techniques become more and more important. Including cognitive rehabilitation, caregiver support, and pharmaceutical and non-pharmacological therapies improves the overall care given to patients and their families.

Vascular dementia is now recognized as a worldwide health concern, which emphasizes the necessity of cross-border cooperation. The implementation of multinational research projects, cultural competency in care delivery, and a collective dedication to resolving healthcare inequities all serve to enhance the effectiveness and inclusivity of vascular dementia treatment.

Empowering Communities and Increasing Knowledge: It is essential to empower communities and increase awareness of vascular dementia to facilitate early identification, care access, and the removal of stigma related to cognitive decline. Education programs aimed at caregivers, people, and healthcare professionals help create a more knowledgeable community that is better equipped to serve persons who are impacted by vascular dementia.

Advocacy for Policy Changes: To alleviate healthcare access inequities, improve programs for caregiver support, and advance research activities, advocacy for policy changes is crucial. A more supportive environment for people with vascular dementia is created by policy reforms that give priority to prevention initiatives, enhance diagnostic technologies, and guarantee equal access to treatment.